PERSONAL PROTECTIVE EQUIPMENT

FOR DIAGNOSTIC X-RAY USE

Report of a BIR Working Party

June 2014 to January 2016

Authors

Peter A Hiles, Glan Clwyd Hospital, Bodelwyddan, Wales

Helen Hughes, Wrexham Maelor Hospital, Wrexham, Wales

Denise Arthur, Harefield Hospital, Harefield, England

Colin J Martin, University of Glasgow, Scotland

Published by

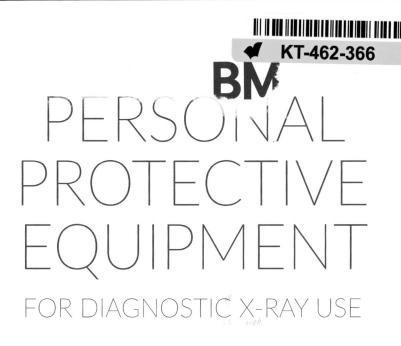

BIR

The British
Institute of
Radiology

The British Institute of Radiology
48–50 St John Street, London EC1M 4DG, UK
www.bir.org.uk
Registered charity number: 215869

Published in the United Kingdom by The British Institute of Radiology, London
© 2016 The Authors and The British Institute of Radiology

British Library Cataloguing in Publication data
A cataloguing record for this publication is available from the British Library

ISBN 978-0-905749-86-0 (Paperback)
ISBN 978-0-905749-84-6 (eBook)

Contents

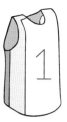

Introduction

In the UK, personal protective equipment (PPE) means:

> "equipment which is intended to be worn or held by a person at work and which protects him against one or more risks to his health or safety".[1]

In the context of this guidance this is confined to equipment intended to be worn by employees in the medical sector to help reduce exposure to diagnostic X-rays. It does not include shielding built into a room and equipment design *e.g.* mobile or articulated screens, or curtains mounted on equipment. PPE should only be used where other methods of protection have not reduced exposures to a level that is as low as reasonably practicable (ALARP) or are not applicable.[2] The aim of this document is to provide practical guidance on the selection, use and maintenance of PPE within the context of medical X-ray usage, with a particular focus on specification, design, fitting, care, quality control and disposal. It therefore has a relevance to a wide range of staff groups in the healthcare sector, particularly those present during X-ray diagnostic, intervention and image guidance procedures.

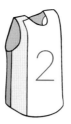

General requirements for PPE

2.1 Legislation, standards and guidance

The International Basic Safety Standard (BSS),[3] European Directive on adoption of BSS[4] and the current UK Ionising Radiations Regulations 1999[5] all require employers to restrict exposure of employees to ionising radiation by, where necessary, providing adequate and suitable PPE. Clear instructions on the use of PPE should be contained within a department's local rules and appropriate storage provided for PPE when it is not being worn. They also require employees to make full and proper use of any PPE provided, report any defects and return PPE to storage after use. Further guidance on these requirements is provided in the accompanying Approved Code of Practice and Guidance[6] and the application to medical radiology is provided in the Medical and Dental Guidance Notes.[7]

In accordance with the Ionising Radiations Regulations[5] Regulation 9, any PPE provided by an employer shall comply with The Personal Protective Equipment at Work Regulations,[1] along with the associated guidance.[8] Employers should also ensure that any PPE they buy bears a "CE" mark and complies with the Personal Protective Equipment Regulations[9] and the European PPE Regulation.[10]

Basically, the employer is required to ensure that any PPE provided is suitable, properly used, stored and maintained and its use properly supervised. This includes conducting a thorough examination at suitable intervals to ensure it remains fit for purpose.

Employers who require employees to handle and wear potentially heavy and uncomfortable PPE, will also need to perform risk assessments as required by the Manual Handling Operations Regulations[11] and the Management of Health and Safety at Work Regulations.[12]

Protective clothing and eyewear, designed for workers undertaking medical X-ray procedures should comply with the requirements of the British Standard BS 61331.[2,13] This standard deals with general requirements such as design, materials used, marking, defining standard sizes and minimum attenuation properties of materials. In particular, the attenuation properties of the protective materials shall be characterized by their values of the attenuation equivalent in defined thicknesses of lead of 0.25 mm, 0.35 mm, 0.5 mm and 1 mm.

2.2 General guidance on selecting PPE

The Personal Protective Equipment at Work Regulations[1] state that:

> "Every employer shall ensure that suitable personal protective equipment is provided to his employees who may be exposed to a risk to their health or safety while at work except where and to the extent that such risk has been adequately controlled by other means which are equally or more effective".

There are a number of occasions when staff are required to remain close to the X-ray tube and/or patient during an X-ray procedure. The purpose of the PPE considered in this guidance is to help keep such occupational exposures from radiation ALARP.[6]

The BSS[3] section 3.95(c) states that:

> "Tasks requiring the use of certain PPE are assigned only to workers who on the basis of medical advice are capable of safely sustaining the extra effort necessary".

A risk assessment should be used to decide on the necessity for and choice and type of PPE, to ensure it is adequate and suitable.[6] In some cases, requiring employees to wear more radiation protective clothing than is essential, could render the wearer liable to other forms of risk alongside that arising from the ionising radiation; for example, the wearing of a lead apron by an employee who is unable to handle or carry its weight without risk of injury. In these circumstances, all reasonable risks need to be balanced in choosing the appropriate PPE.

The BSS[3] section 3.95(e) suggests that:

> "account is taken of any additional exposure that could result owing to the additional time taken or the inconvenience, and of any non-radiological risks that might be associated with using PPE while performing the task".

In choosing between the different designs of PPE the wearer and conditions of use should be considered. Wearing an excessively heavy apron can cause discomfort and may even prolong the examination. It may be necessary to reduce the weight to achieve comfort and reduce any associated health risks. It is recommended that PPE is trialled before purchase to ensure suitability for local requirements and practice.

Factors to consider when determining whether PPE is suitable include: the physical effort required to do the job, the posture to be adopted, how long the PPE must be worn, the work environment, the health of the person wearing the PPE and its impact on their movement when performing the required tasks. One important case to be considered would be pregnant staff. The aim should be to choose PPE which will give maximum protection to the foetus while ensuring minimum discomfort to the wearer, as uncomfortable equipment is unlikely to be worn properly and can increase fatigue. There have also been reports linking the long-term wearing of lead aprons with an increased incidence of back pain.[14] The PPE should be chosen to provide the degree of user protection required by foreseeable conditions of use without leading to an increase in exposure time as a result of impedance of user gestures, posture or movement. In the specific context of healthcare, consideration will also need to be given to the fact that in many situations the scattered radiation field that employees may be required to enter is spatially and temporally non-uniform, with radiation potentially coming from a variety of different directions and may be switched on and off a number of times during a medical procedure.

Those who are required to regularly wear PPE are usually best placed to know what is involved, and they should be consulted and involved in the selection and specification of the PPE. There is a better chance of PPE being used effectively if it is accepted by each wearer.

There will be considerable differences in the physical dimensions of different workers and therefore more than one type or size of PPE may be needed. It would also be useful to have monograms on the PPE to aid identification in such cases.

In selecting PPE, the employer should consult a Radiation Protection Adviser (RPA) for advice on restricting exposure and appointed safety representative(s) regarding the suitability of PPE for the wearer.[6]

Appendix 1 provides a summary table of suggested PPE requirements for a range of applications. However, a decision on local requirements should be subject to a risk assessment and other considerations highlighted above.

Appendix 2 provides a framework for conducting such a risk assessment.

2.3 Information, instruction and training of employees

Where an employer is required to ensure that PPE is provided to an employee, the employer shall also ensure that the employee is provided with such information, instruction and training as is adequate and appropriate to enable the employee to make effective use of the PPE. For example:

a. Explain the risks and why PPE is needed.

b. Provide instructions on the proper use of PPE, how to correctly fit and wear it and any manual handling issues.

c. Explain related issues of infection control that need to be addressed in the healthcare environment.

d. Indicate how to store it, clean it and recognize defects, damage and wear.

In addition, it is recommended that the employer provides a suitable number of trained advisers to instruct employees on the correct way to wear PPE.

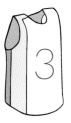

Effectiveness of PPE

In choosing a lead equivalence, the attenuation of scattered radiation is assumed to be essentially the same as that of the primary (incident) beam and this provides a margin of safety.

In determining the level of protection required, consideration needs to be given not only to the stochastic risk (cancer induction and hereditary effects) but also tissue reactions (deterministic effects) and the radiosensitivity of the eye lens.[15] These are incorporated into the dose limits[4,5] and the application of ALARP.

3.1 Transmission data and dose reduction

Measuring the radiation (air kerma) transmitted through PPE in order to assess its effectiveness as a shielding material would appear to be relatively simple. However, historically such transmission measurements have been performed using narrow, primary X-ray quality beams, whereas in clinical practice the vast majority of staff are subject to broad beam secondary (scattered) radiation.[16]

In addition, the transmission of non-lead materials (**Section 3.3**) varies with the X-ray beam energy in a different way to lead. For most medical X-ray applications the tube voltage range is from 60 to 120 kV, which corresponds to mean energies of approximately 35 to 60 keV. At these energies the photoelectric effect dominates the X-ray absorption and the choice of protective material must take into account the k-edge absorption of its individual components, where radiation of energies immediately above the edge are strongly absorbed. For example, the attenuation factor for tin, a material used in lead-free aprons, is less than lead at 60 kV but similar at 120 kV. This means that to properly characterize a material as equivalent to a certain thickness of lead, the specification should state the applicable range of X-ray beam energies.[14,17-19]

These two issues have led to a new standard for specifying lead equivalence of protective clothing,[13] which requires measurement under broad-beam conditions and specifying the range of radiation qualities over which the lead equivalence applies.

As previously stated, the purpose of the PPE is to help keep occupational exposures from radiation within applicable dose limits,[5] which are defined in terms of the effective dose to the person who may be irradiated.[15] However, radiation is generally measured in terms of air kerma. So that, whilst increasing any shielding will lower both the transmitted air kerma and the effective dose, the ratio of these dose quantities will vary with the energy spectrum of the X-ray beam. Nevertheless, in the energy range used for diagnostic radiology, air kerma generally represents a reasonable overestimate of the effective dose, especially when compared with using personal dose monitor results [usually quoted in terms of personal dose equivalent, $H_p(10)$].[20]

3.2 Combining PPE

In deciding on the appropriate level of protection, all available PPE should be considered. For instance, it has been shown that the combination of a 0.25 mm lead apron with a thyroid collar results in a greater reduction in effective dose than does increasing the lead apron thickness to 0.35 mm or even 0.5 mm.[21,22] This is because, as the lead apron thickness is increased beyond 0.25 mm, the effective dose is dominated by contributions from unprotected organs in the head and neck. To illustrate this further, published attenuation data[23] and PCXMC dose calculation software[24] have been used to model an anterior–posterior (AP) whole body irradiation in order to estimate the effective dose saving from different combinations of PPE in **Figure 1**. This shows that when wearing a 0.25 mm lead apron, using 75 kV X-rays, adding a thyroid collar will halve the effective dose, whereas increasing the thickness of lead in the apron to 0.35 mm will only decrease it by 10%. This simple model demonstrates the impact of combining PPE, but it

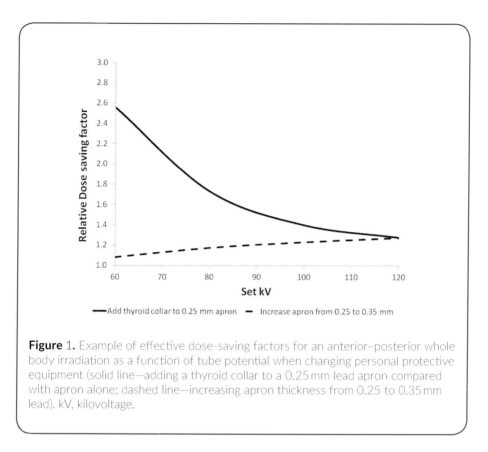

Figure 1. Example of effective dose-saving factors for an anterior–posterior whole body irradiation as a function of tube potential when changing personal protective equipment (solid line—adding a thyroid collar to a 0.25 mm lead apron compared with apron alone; dashed line—increasing apron thickness from 0.25 to 0.35 mm lead). kV, kilovoltage.

should be noted that the actual effective dose to operators and the protection provided by the lead apron vary significantly with irradiation conditions.[25]

However, the effective dose saving does not give the complete picture since it is known that the cancer induction risk for the thyroid rapidly decreases with age and females are more susceptible than males. So, using the same model used to produce **Figure 1** and published risk factors,[26] the relative saving in cancer induction risk has been estimated for a 20-year-old and 40-year-old female. The result (**Figure 2** top) for the 20 year old shows a similar trend to the dose saving in **Figure 1**, particularly below 100 kV. Whereas, for the 40 year old (**Figure 2** bottom) the value of adding a thyroid collar over increasing the apron thickness has diminished. This simple modelling is indicative, although it does not account for any additional shielding provided by a collar, of tissues at the top of the chest not covered by an apron.

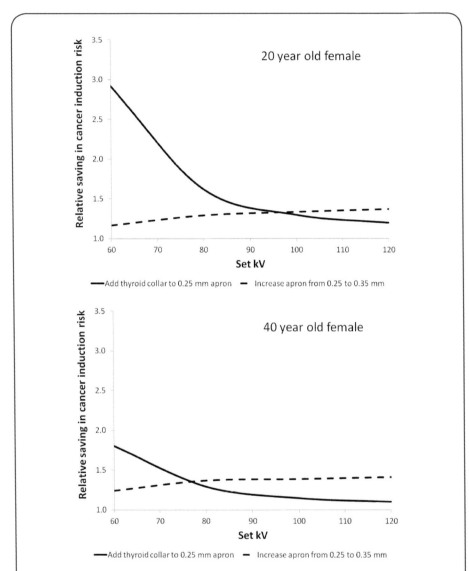

Figure 2. Example of cancer induction risk-saving factors for an anterior–posterior whole body irradiation as a function of tube potential when changing personal protective equipment (solid line—adding a thyroid collar to a 0.25 mm lead apron compared with apron alone; dashed line—increasing apron thickness from 0.25 to 0.35 mm lead), for a 20-year-old female (top) and 40-year-old female (bottom). kV, kilovoltage.

Thus it is important that younger female staff are alerted to the importance of wearing a thyroid collar, but also that the burden of wearing a heavy apron should be balanced with the introduction of a thyroid collar, for example, by only requiring a 0.35 mm apron to be worn alongside a collar for situations where equipment is regularly operating at high kilovoltages.

3.3 Lead and lead-free materials

In the past, protective aprons and coverings have been manufactured from lead powder-loaded polymer or elastomer sheets. However, in a drive to reduce the overall weight of material and address the issue of disposal of lead aprons as toxic waste, new materials have been introduced.[18] These new materials can be either totally lead-free or combined with lead in so called "light-weight lead" composites and are designed to provide the same attenuation as an equivalent thickness of lead at less weight.[14]

Similar levels of attenuation can be achieved with lighter aprons because the alternative metals are more efficient per unit mass than lead for absorbing X-ray photons with energies between 40 keV and 88 keV. These aprons may be more effective for attenuating scattered X-rays generated at 70–80 kV, but less effective above 100 kV.[27] The combining of low and high atomic number (Z) metals, in so-called bilayer materials, can overcome some of these limitations and result in improved attenuation properties, at lighter weight, compared with lead.[28] They provide a reasonable alternative where weight reduction is required, for example to alleviate back problems.

Lightweight or "lead-free" aprons have different X-ray transmission properties for different X-ray spectra compared with traditional lead aprons. Nevertheless, attenuation properties are often quoted by manufacturers in terms of lead equivalence and this can be misleading (**Section 3.1**). For this reason considerable care is required in assessing lead-free protective aprons. Experimental measurements of transmission for comparisons of attenuation should use broadband X-ray beams and involve different X-ray spectra. They should concentrate on beam energies used clinically in the facility where the aprons will be worn.

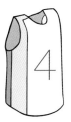

Aprons and tunics

Apron refers to PPE designed to protect the trunk of the body from scattered radiation arising from the X-ray tube and the patient. Aprons should be worn when employees are required to work outside a fixed protective screen and in close proximity to a patient during an X-ray exposure. They should be so designed that they can be put on and taken off without assistance and staff should be encouraged to remove aprons between cases or at the end of a session if they can be removed without undue manual effort.

4.1 Design

These come in three basic forms (**Figure 3**): a tabard, an apron and two-piece apron. The generic term "apron" used in the following sections is intended to cover all three.

Tabard. These consist of two panels either joined at both shoulders with a head opening or joined at one shoulder with a clip fastening at the other shoulder. Fastenings are also provided to draw the material together at the sides.

Apron. These are made up of three panels and can fasten at the sides or "wrap-around" the wearer. They are designed to distribute the weight through straps, shoulder flaps and, occasionally, by a belt.

Two-piece apron. These consist of a vest and a wrap-over kilt, distributing the weight between the wearer's shoulders and hips. Dividing the weight between the two pieces can also reduce the manual handling required when putting the garments on.

Backless aprons can be purchased to reduce weight but run the risk of exposure of unprotected areas of the body.

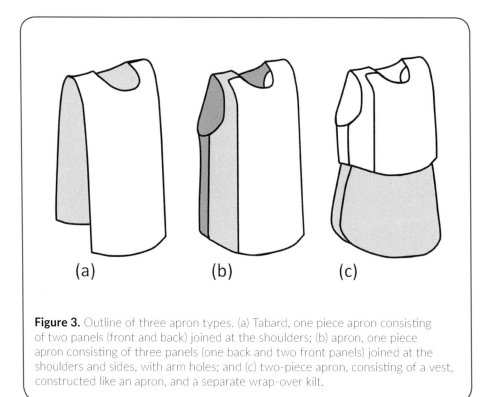

Figure 3. Outline of three apron types. (a) Tabard, one piece apron consisting of two panels (front and back) joined at the shoulders; (b) apron, one piece apron consisting of three panels (one back and two front panels) joined at the shoulders and sides, with arm holes; and (c) two-piece apron, consisting of a vest, constructed like an apron, and a separate wrap-over kilt.

4.2 Specification and selection

When providing a protective apron it is worth emphasising to employees that, where changing position is practicable, they can reduce their effective dose by approximately a factor of 2 if they move 30 cm away from the side of the patient when exposing. This is a far greater reduction than may be achieved by increasing lead apron thickness from 0.25 mm to 0.5 mm.[29]

Owing to the wide range of differences in design and manufacture, it is important to understand the specification when selecting aprons. To illustrate this, consider the following example. When selecting a 0.25 mm wrap-around apron, it is generally assumed that this provides 0.5 mm lead protection at the front (anterior) where the panels overlap,[30] but this is not necessarily the case. The manufacturer may reduce the overall weight of the apron by making the combination of wrap-over material equal to 0.25 mm lead, thus meeting the specification but with obvious implications on correct fitting and wearing of the apron. It is unfortunate that current guidance on PPE specification[2] does not require manufacturers to label individual panels, at least for situations where they differ in attenuation within the same garment.

The Medical & Dental Guidance Notes,[7] paragraph 3.119, states that,

> "Body aprons should be available with a protective equivalent of not less than 0.25 mm lead for use with X-rays up to 100 kV and not less than 0.35 mm lead for use with X-rays over 100 kV".

An international standard on PPE[2] defines four different categories of protective aprons, depending on workload and apron design (**Table 1**).

Table 1. Suggested apron protection with workload for two different apron designs,[2] where, in this British Standard, "closed" means, in addition to front protection offered by an "open" apron, the design includes protecting the sides of the body from not more than 10 cm below the armpit to the knees

Apron category	Description	Lead equivalent (mm Pb)
L	Light-duty protective apron	≥0.25 over entire area
H	Heavy-duty protective aprons	≥0.35 for the front section and ≥0.25 for the remaining parts
LC	Light-duty closed protective aprons	≥0.25 over the entire area
HC	Heavy-duty closed protective aprons	≥0.35 for the front section and ≥0.25 for the remaining parts

For procedures performed on small patients and children, the scattered radiation is less and so the thickness of lead protection can be reduced compared with larger, adult patients.[30] However, this is generally impractical except in specialist paediatric centres, since there is the risk that in having a range of apron thicknesses the wrong one could be chosen.

See **Appendix 1** for a summary table of suggested PPE requirements for a range of applications. However, a decision on local requirements should be subject to a risk assessment and other considerations highlighted in **Sections 2.2** and **3.2** above (see also **Appendix 2**).

Some newer aprons are designed to be lightweight while maintaining lead equivalence (**Section 3.3**). The heavy weight of some aprons can pose a problem for employees who have to wear them for extended periods of time. There are reports of back injuries associated with staff wearing their lead aprons for many years.[14] However, this may be due to the general recommendation in the USA for interventional X-ray staff to wear 0.5 mm lead aprons,[14] which is uncommon in the UK.

For pregnant employees the aim should be to ensure the foetal dose is less than the specified dose limit (currently 1 mSv) during the declared term of the pregnancy.[5] When an apron needs to be worn then it is important to ensure correct fitting to protect the foetus for the duration of the pregnancy. This is particularly important for tabard style aprons with a side opening.

Choosing an apron is a balance between a good fit and the weight of the apron, where the weight of an apron depends on the selected size and lead equivalence. A modern, medium size apron can weigh between 4.5 and 6 kg and a combined vest/kilt can weigh approximately 1 kg more than a similar one piece apron. The difference in weight between a 0.25 mm and 0.35 mm lead apron can be around 1.5 kg. However, examples have been found where an older 0.25 mm lead apron weighs more than a modern 0.35 mm lead apron.

Staff who may not be able to bear the weight of an apron might wish to consider alternatives such as an apron suspension system[31] or floor mounted radiation protection cabinet,[32,33] which can also offer protection for head/eyes.

When specifying aprons it is also important to stipulate the outer coating required. For example, they should be waterproof and wipeable, and in some cases, with antibacterial coating.

4.3 Fitting

Lead aprons are available in different sizes, so in selecting an apron, it is important to make sure that there is a good fit. A tailored or correctly fitting garment is very important for protection, comfort and perception of weight. In fact it has been reported that the fit of the apron is often more important in limiting staff dose than the thickness of lead.[22] Employees should therefore be suitably trained and, where applicable, required to wear and fasten all parts of an apron.

A suggested procedure for putting on an apron is shown below:

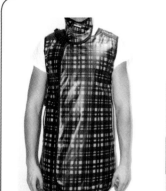

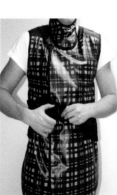

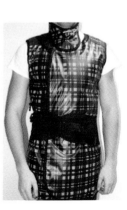

1 Put coat on and fasten velcro fastener so that both sides are completely covered and wrap over is parallel with the line of the body.

2 Shrug your shoulders to take the weight of the apron off the back. Adjust the lumbar support belt. The belt should be pulled snugly but not crease the apron.

3 Release your shoulders and the weight of the apron will now be on the shoulders and hips and not the back.

Aprons should cover at least from the suprasternal notch to just above the knees, front and back, and include the shoulders. It is suggested that the depth of the arm holes should not exceed 100 mm below the armpit to ensure adequate protection of breast tissue. Some manufacturers provide separate patterns for aprons for male and female use, where the female version has smaller arm holes for more effective breast protection. The height of the neckline should be such as to ensure adequate coverage of the chest and sternum. According to the British Standard BS EN 61331-3,[2] the width of the material on each shoulder shall not be less than 8 cm for persons having the minimum chest girth of 76 cm and shall be increased as chest girth increases.

If two overlaid layers are needed to meet lead-equivalent requirement (**Section 4.2**), ensure the overlap is sufficient and the wearers are fully aware of the need to completely overlap the panels.

Kilts can be constructed of one or two panels. In the latter case care should be taken since the panels may gape if the wrong size is chosen. Also a sufficient overlap (for example 50 mm) is required between the kilt and vest to maintain adequate protection, especially as the wearer moves to perform required tasks.

Ideally a department will have a selection of sizes and types so that wearers can find some degree of comfort and personal preference. If staff members are wearing their PPE for a large part of their working day, a risk assessment should be performed (**Section 2.2** and **Appendix 2**) to determine if personalized garments should be provided. In some cases this may mean being made-to-measure, but the rewards of personal comfort and the individual's willingness to care for their garments may make this worthwhile. It may be possible to have a light-weight back of 0.25 mm lead equivalence and a heavier front of 0.35 mm lead equivalence, depending upon workload. Monograms can also be added to aid identification.

Belts are effective in distributing weight and should be encouraged. Some designs include an internal belt and this can be particularly effective in relieving the weight on the back, neck and shoulders.

Those wearing a lead apron should also be aware that any external pocket on an apron is generally not protected, so it is not suitable to house radiosensitive items (*e.g.* personal dosimeters when not in use).

Examples to illustrate the correct wearing of PPE and some common mistakes are shown in **Figures 4–12**.

Tops

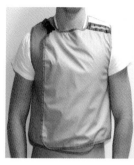

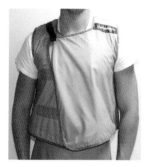

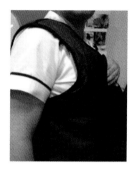

Figure 4. Correctly fitting top of two piece apron.

Figure 5. Incorrectly fitting top of two piece apron. Velcro fastening should be completely closed to facilitate the correct lead protection across the chest.

Figure 6. Poor fit, arm holes are too large, which could result in increased breast tissue exposure.

Kilts

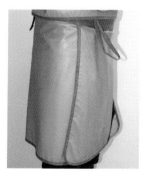

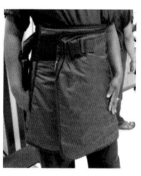

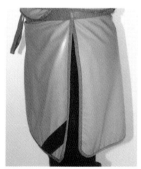

Figure 7. Correctly fitting panelled kilt.

Figure 8. Very poor fit of kilt that should overlap seam to seam. The area not overlapping at the front in this case is only 0.15 mm lead equivalent. The belt is also not fastened properly.

Figure 9. Incorrectly fitting panelled kilt showing gap between panels that should overlap.

Single and two piece aprons

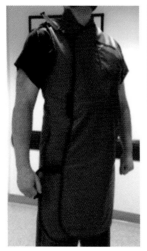 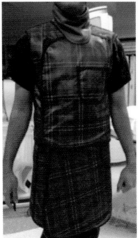 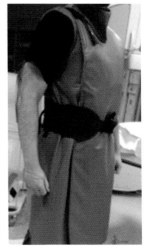

Figure 10. Good fitting coat with inside belt (lumbar support).

Figure 11. Good fitting top and kilt but thyroid collar is too large and so is creased in use, which could lead to cracking.

Figure 12. Apron too big causing folding and creasing at waist.

4.4 Care and storage

Since protective aprons are constructed from layers of metal powder-loaded polymer sheets bound together[18] they are relatively fragile and should be cared for properly to maintain the designed protective benefit for as long as possible. Apart from deterioration due to ageing, lead aprons can be damaged by incorrect handling, storage or placing near a source of heat, such as a radiator and direct sunlight, and very cold areas such as close to air conditioning units. Users can damage the aprons when they are wearing them by resting their hands in the arm holes, which can lead to stretching, or sitting with the apron tucked up under them, which can cause cracks to develop.

A lead apron tends to crack when folded or laid over a pointed object. When not in use, aprons should be hung carefully on designated hangers or wrapped over a rail or reinforced bar.

Aprons and vests should be hung by both shoulders to distribute the weight evenly. Kilts can be stored on rails or on hangers. When hanging a kilt both waistband straps must be used to spread the weight and prevent creasing and stress cracks.

For general advice on cleaning and infection control see **Section 9.2**. In some clinical environments it is preferable to wear a plastic apron on top of the apron to make cleaning easier.

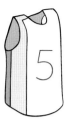

Thyroid collars

The thyroid gland has been highlighted as a particularly radiosensitive organ,[15] but lead aprons do not protect the head and neck. Therefore, employees who are likely to be subject to high levels of scattered radiation directed towards the head and neck should wear a thyroid collar. If no thyroid protection is worn, the dose to the unprotected thyroid can lead to a doubling of the effective dose.

Since the relative sensitivity of the thyroid gland to radiation-induced cancer is strongly biased towards younger people (male <30 years, female <40 years) and there is a longer time for any induced cancer to manifest itself, it is particularly important to consider this age group when deciding if thyroid collars are required.[14]

5.1 Design and specification

Thyroid collars come as one or two lengths of material, similar to that used for aprons, which is fastened at the back of the neck. They should cover the front half of the neck, including the thyroid gland and should extend from under the jaw down to the neckline of the protective apron (**Figure 13**).

The reduction in equivalent dose to the thyroid by a protective collar is likely to be a factor of 10–12 for a collar containing 0.5 mm lead and 5–7 for a 0.35 mm lead collar.[22]

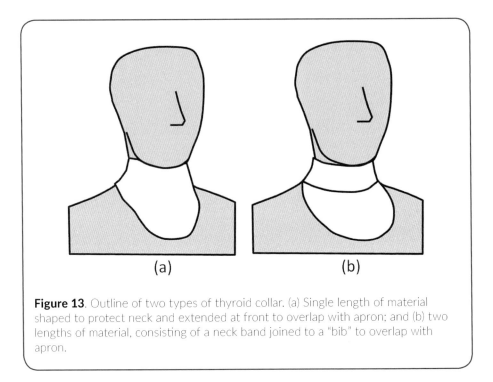

Figure 13. Outline of two types of thyroid collar. (a) Single length of material shaped to protect neck and extended at front to overlap with apron; and (b) two lengths of material, consisting of a neck band joined to a "bib" to overlap with apron.

For interventional procedures it is recommended that a thyroid collar incorporating 0.35 or 0.5 mm of lead, depending on workload, should always be worn. It has been suggested[34] that:

"thyroid protection is necessary for all personnel whose personal monitor readings at the collar level (unshielded) exceed 4 mSv [$H_p(10)$] in a month".

The authors of this guide consider this rather high as this could give a contribution of 2 mSv to the annual effective dose from the thyroid, as well as 1 mSv from the brain and salivary glands. It is therefore suggested that if the annual thyroid equivalent dose exceeds 7 mSv then a thyroid collar should be worn.

5.2 Fitting

Thyroid collars can be made of rigid or soft material and either straight or curved in shape. The design and length of the selected collar can depend on the length of neck, for instance the neck band and bib-style collar may suit smaller necks.

A quick reference guide to wearing a thyroid collar is shown below:

Indicates the position of the thyroid gland which should be fully covered by the protective collar.

It is worth bearing in mind that some thyroid collars have no lead protection at the back, therefore it is important to have the deepest part at the front and centre, ensuring the area of the thyroid is adequately covered.

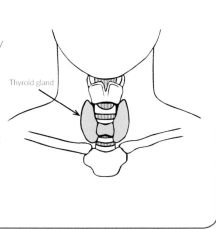

Thyroid gland

The shield should be close fitting to the neck, high enough to cover the thyroid and low enough at the front to overlap with the protective apron or top.

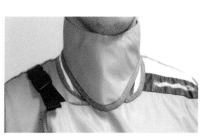

A selection of different designs may be required as the needs of people with differing length necks will impact on comfort and therefore correct fitting and protective qualities.

Too loose a thyroid shield can lead to an unacceptable gap between the shield and the neck where the thyroid does not have good coverage. Too low a thyroid shield will have the same effect.

Thyroid collars fasten at the back by a strip of velcro. Velcro fastenings can become "clogged" resulting in ineffective closure and should be "de-fluffed" regularly to maintain effectiveness.

The effectiveness of a thyroid collar is dependent on its being worn correctly. For instance, it has been estimated that if a collar is worn loosely for comfort, leaving the upper thyroid unprotected, it can halve the effective protection factor.[22]

Comfort is also important since they may need to be worn for extended periods. Thus when purchasing collars, it is important to consider the softness of the material and bear in mind that the level of comfort is not necessarily related to the cost of the item.

Example images of how to wear and how not to wear thyroid collars are shown in **Figures 14–16**.

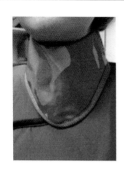 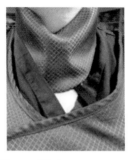 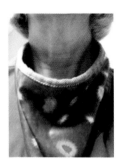

Figure 14. Good-fitting thyroid collar with suitable overlap with apron.

Figure 15. Poor-fitting apron leaving gap between apron and (poor-fitting) thyroid collar.

Figure 16. Thyroid collar too big and so fails to cover and protect thyroid.

5.3 Care and storage

Since these collars are made of a similar material to lead aprons, similar care and storage requirements to those outlined in **Sections 4.4** and **9** apply.

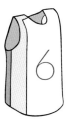

Eye shields

Recent research has concluded that the eye lens is more sensitive to ionising radiation than had previously been thought, and this has led to a recommendation that the dose limit for the eye lens be reduced to 20 mSv per annum from its current level of 150 mSv per annum.[3,4,35] The new dose limit will come into effect in the UK from 2018. Radiation doses to the lens of the eye from scattered radiation for some employees, including but not exclusively, interventional radiologists and cardiologists with high workloads, can exceed this limit, unless appropriate radiation protection measures are put in place.[36]

Therefore the need to consider eye protection has taken on greater importance. Lead glasses can provide a key component of the protection against scattered radiation. For instance, a study of interventional cardiologists in France reports that the risk of developing posterior sub-capsular (PSC) opacities can be significantly decreased by regular use of protective lead glasses.[37]

Eye doses are influenced by tube angulation, operator position and beam collimation. The operator usually stands adjacent to the patient couch, often to the side of the X-ray tube/image receptor gantry. When a clinician is carrying out a procedure, he/she will be viewing the resulting images on the monitor while X-rays are being produced rather than looking towards the patient. Thus the operator's eyes will be irradiated from below and from the side, so it is important to protect the eye lens against irradiation from these directions (**Figure 17**). Other staff in the vicinity may also require eye protection.

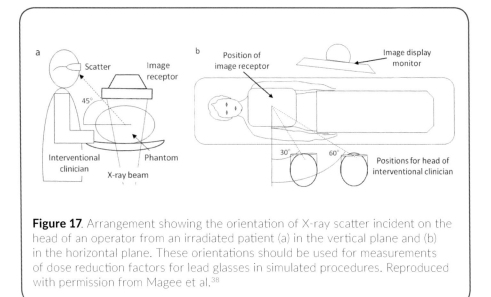

Figure 17. Arrangement showing the orientation of X-ray scatter incident on the head of an operator from an irradiated patient (a) in the vertical plane and (b) in the horizontal plane. These orientations should be used for measurements of dose reduction factors for lead glasses in simulated procedures. Reproduced with permission from Magee et al.[38]

The proximity to the eyes of patient tissue on which unattenuated X-rays are incident is a major factor in determining the residual dose to the eye lens when protective eyewear is worn. For exposures from the front, differences between various categories of glasses relate to the sizes of the lenses, and so the proximity of unprotected and therefore irradiated tissue. For exposures from the side, the eye dose depends on the closeness of the fit to the facial contours and the extent of the protection from the side. When the scattered radiation is incident from below, radiation may enter not only from the side, but also through the gaps underneath the glass lenses.

6.1 Design and specification

Protective eyewear includes eyeglasses or goggles and transparent shields, visors or masks that fit on the operator's head. The general impression is that such eyewear is significantly heavier than normal eye glasses. However, modern designs and fabrication mean that it is possible to get comfortable, well-fitting eyewear weighing as little as 60 g.

A variety of lead glasses are available. A close fit to the facial contours, particularly around the underside, can be as important as the lead equivalence, in order to ensure that protection against exposures from below and to the side is adequate. Wraparound glasses with angled front lenses provide good protection for radiation incident from the side and below because they fit more snugly to the facial contours and so the gaps between the frames and head tend to be smaller. Conventionally designed glasses with large front lenses and side shields are also a good option (**Figure 18**).

Lead glasses, designed to fit over conventional spectacles are available, but are bulky, and have larger gaps underneath. The dose reduction is often less for irradiation from the side due to the larger spaces left between the lead glasses and the head for the prescription spectacles.[38] If the head is angled towards an image display monitor, which is likely to be the case for the majority of the time, then scattered radiation is able to pass through gaps behind the lead glasses to irradiate the eyes directly. Close-fitting prescription lead glasses provide a better option for sight correction in most circumstances, even though, depending on the prescription, they can be relatively expensive and could only be used by the individual staff member.

The majority of protective glasses have lenses with protection equivalent to 0.75 mm or 0.5 mm of lead and many have protection in side shields of 0.5 mm or 0.35 mm lead equivalence. The lower value of lead equivalence in the lenses often offers good protection, and the fit and size of the lens are more important than the difference between 0.75 mm and 0.5 mm lead protection.

It is important to check that critical parts of the frames are protected, as some models, particularly the heavier "fit-over" glasses, do not use protection in the

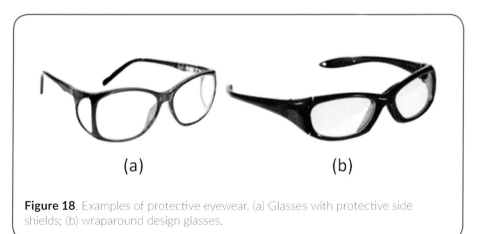

(a)   (b)

Figure 18. Examples of protective eyewear. (a) Glasses with protective side shields; (b) wraparound design glasses.

frames and side-arm in order to keep the weight down, but this will leave gaps in protection at critical positions.

Curved face shields of lower lead equivalence (0.1 mm lead), held in place by a headband offer an alternative, and provide as good protection as the glasses. These cover the whole of the face and so also reduce the exposure of regions of the head surrounding the eyes that would make a significant contribution to the eye dose from X-rays scattered within the facial tissues.[38] However, it is important for staff to try these out for acceptability.

The protection to the eyes provided by protective eyewear can be quantified in terms of dose reduction factors (DRFs), which is the ratio of the dose with no protection, divided by that when protection is used. DRFs between 5 and 10 have been reported from experimental measurements for a variety of lead glasses when protecting against X-rays incident from the front in the same horizontal plane as the eyes.[39-41] However, the protection provided in practice depends on the angle at which scatter from the X-ray equipment and patient is incident on the head. Custom-designed lead glasses with a lead equivalence of 0.75 mm provide DRFs between 3.5 and 6,[14,38,40,41] and 0.50 mm lead equivalence pairs provide DRFs of 3–4.

It is suggested that protective eyewear is considered when staff eye lens equivalent doses are likely to exceed 6 mSv per annum and is recommended when doses exceed 10 mSv per annum, unless alternative protective measures (e.g. ceiling suspended shield) are able to reduce doses.[42]

6.2 Fitting

Protective glasses are provided in a range of different frame designs. Operators should be given the opportunity to try out different options. Employees are often required to wear the glasses for a significant length of time and also regularly turn their head to view displayed images (e.g. interventional radiology or cardiology). Therefore, proper fit and side protection are very important.

Face shields provide an alternative to protective glasses for those who wish to wear their ordinary prescription glasses or if splash protection is also needed. It is important that these are tried out during a procedure, as some users have reported that the face shields have a tendency to mist up.

The use of protective eyewear has to be balanced against any impeding of movement, physical discomfort or impaired vision that may be experienced whilst wearing the device. In addition, poorly designed or heavy glasses can slip down the nose which is distracting and can interfere with the procedure. Adjustable headbands on the arms of the glasses should be used to prevent this.

6.3 Care and storage

Lead glass lenses are soft and easily scratched and damaged by some cleaning fluids. Cleaning can be carried out with warm soapy water. It is advisable to keep them in their protective cases to prevent scratching of the lenses.

6.4 Issues with measuring eye lens dose

Personal dosemeters for measurement of eye doses will not take account of the protection provided by the eyewear. Measurements of the protection offered by lead glasses can provide useful data based on which adjustments to dosemeter reading values recorded by unshielded eye dosemeters can be made, in order to derive a dose representing that to the lens of the eye. The measurements for any glasses should take account of directions of exposure encountered in clinical practice (**Figure 17**), and the measurement technique and the results should be documented. Generally the DRF applied should not be >4. Where no measurements are available to confirm the DRF, but the glasses are of approved design, a factor of 2 represents a conservative approach to account for the protection offered.[38]

A DRF should only be applied if the employee wears the protective eyewear and dosemeters consistently for all work with ionising radiation. Appropriate supervision and quality assurance measures must be in place with regular documented checks to confirm that the employee always wears the protective eyewear.

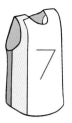

Hand protection

For some procedures the hands of operators can be close to the X-ray beam. If the hands stray into the primary beam significant doses can be received from very short exposure times.

In the case of interventional procedures, the position of the operator's hands relative to the patient access point can have a substantial effect on the dose level. Percutaneous procedures such as biliary drainage and stent placement require the operator to manipulate catheters inserted close to the area being imaged and this can give relatively high doses to the finger tips.[43] In the majority of cases the operator stands next to the X-ray tube, the non-dominant hand will hold the catheter close to the edge of the X-ray field, while the dominant hand performs manipulations.

7.1 Design and specification

Generally protective gloves are designed simply to protect the hands from scattered radiation. These may be in the form of disposable surgical gloves incorporating some lead equivalence. The level of protection is generally small,[14] for example, ranging from <0.02 mm up to around 0.07 mm lead equivalence. Operators wearing such gloves can get a false sense of security and fail to take all necessary precautions to keep finger doses ALARP. If a hand protected by a glove strays into the X-ray field, depending on position, the dose rate may increase automatically to compensate for the attenuation, thereby negating any attempt to reduce radiation dose to the hand and increasing the radiation dose to the patient.

For procedures in which the hands and forearms need to be protected whilst very close to the radiation beam or in areas of high scatter, protective gloves should have a lead equivalence of at least 0.25 mm lead.[2]

Provided finger doses are likely to be well below 150 mSv, hand protection is generally not used and distance and handling tools are used to keep doses ALARP.

7.2 Fitting

Gloves need to provide sufficient flexibility to allow the operator to perform the required hand manipulations with ease, since a reduction in dexterity can lead to fatigue and prolonged examinations. In some cases sterile lead gloves may need to be provided.

7.3 Care and storage

Sterile gloves are single use only and disposed of in clinical waste.

Lead gloves/gauntlets, such as those used in fluoroscopy, should be kept, checked and cleaned in the same way as other PPE (**Sections 4.4** and **9**).

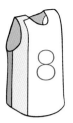

Other protective equipment

This section provides a brief outline of other forms of protective equipment, some of which is not strictly PPE, but is closely associated with PPE.

8.1 Leg shields

When the X-ray tube is positioned below the couch, the primary beam is scattered back downwards, so unprotected legs can receive a significant dose *e.g.* 2.6 mSv per procedure.[44] Where there is no table side shield, radiation dose to the legs can be greater than those to the hands. The dose to the feet of operators is closely related to the kerma-area product (KAP) when no protection is used, with procedures having a KAP of 100 Gy cm^2 giving a dose to the legs of about 1 mGy.[44]

Before considering additional PPE for the feet, the operator should first be encouraged to take a step back from the couch during exposures.

Leg shields (shin pad type), used in conjunction with other PPE, may be useful, especially if mobile or table side shielding is not available. These are similar to cricket pads with adjustable fastenings to provide a comfortable fit along the length of the leg. In order to ensure suitable coverage of the lower limbs it may be necessary to have a variety of sizes. Care should be the same as outlined for lead aprons in **Section 4**. Since it has been shown[44] that the level of dose depends on the type and complexity of the procedure and the equipment used, local monitoring is recommended to determine if leg shields are required. It has been suggested[45] that if the annual dose to the operator's legs exceeds 50 mSv then protective measures should be put in place.

8.2 Surgical cap

For X-ray procedures where staff are positioned "sideways" on to the X-ray equipment and/or patient, the "closest" side of the operator may receive significantly more scattered radiation. In the case of cardiovascular catheterization, one report suggests that a KAP of 6000 Gy cm^2 gives a maximum dose to the side of the head closest to the equipment/patient of approximately 1 mGy.[46] Doses will depend on the operator's height and head angle in relation to the equipment and patient.

Disposable surgical caps made of lightweight (<150 g), lead equivalent protective material with adjustable cloth covering are available and have been shown to be effective in reducing the radiation dose to the operator's head.[46,47]

8.3 Drapes

Sterile protective drapes, though not strictly PPE, can reduce radiation dose to the eyes and hands of operators when used correctly.[48] The drapes are generally single use items. It is essential that these are kept out of the primary radiation beam or the automatic exposure controls for the fluoroscopy unit may drive exposure factors up to compensate for the reduction in radiation reaching the image detector and thus causing an increase in patient and staff dose.

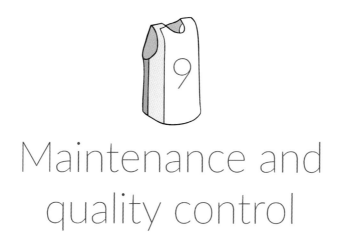

Maintenance and quality control

Suppliers of PPE should provide information and instructions on use, storage, cleaning, disinfection and maintenance.[11] This section is intended to supplement such information and provide additional practical guidance.

9.1 General care and storage

PPE can be relatively fragile and should be cared for properly to maintain the designed protective benefit for as long as possible. Apart from deterioration due to ageing, lead aprons can be damaged by incorrect handling, storage or placing near a source of heat, such as a radiator and direct sunlight, and very cold areas, such as close to air conditioning units.

Proper storage of lead aprons is important to maintain the integrity of the lead. A variety of storage systems, both fixed and freestanding are available. Consideration should be given to:

- how many items are to be kept in a particular location

- the type of PPE used

- should the storage be mobile or fixed?

- is the storage to be central or distributed throughout various clinical areas?

If PPE are removed for a short period, perhaps between cases, then storing it flat *e.g.* on a table top is acceptable. Never fold PPE or leave in a heap on the floor.

A rail with hangers can cause problems when the rail is full and items are placed over the top. The sharper ends of the hanger hooks can make small holes in the delicate protective material but not necessarily damage the outer cover sufficiently to make the damage apparent.

Lead aprons are heavy and cumbersome and so the height of the hanger can have an effect of the level of manual handling required. Careful design of hangers could also aid the handling and putting on of an apron. It is important to ensure that the apron storage can support the required number of the aprons (which can weigh in excess of 100 kg) and that sufficient hangers are available to prevent multi-loading of aprons on a single hanger. It may also be necessary to provide suitable hangers to accommodate kilts and thyroid collars.

Small items such as thyroid collars and belts may be stored in baskets or on shelves or wrapped around a horizontal rail.

Any storage that is overloaded could result in some of the PPE being crushed and damaged. Storage fixed to walls can become so overloaded that their acceptable weight limit is exceeded and they fall down.

Fixed and mobile storage is available and how and where the PPE is used should be considered in deciding the most appropriate form of storage. For example, mobile rails may be more suitable where aprons are shared between several rooms such as in theatres.

Inappropriate use of some storage may itself lead to damage of the garments.

Examples of how to store and how not to store PPE are given in **Figures 19–25**.

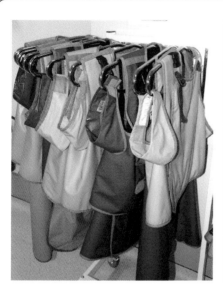 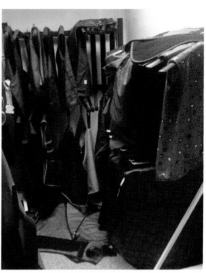

Figure 19. Illustrates aprons and thyroid collars correctly stored on hangers.

Figure 20. Illustrates that even when you have good storage it may not be used correctly.

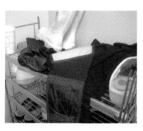 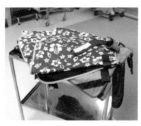 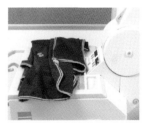

Figure 21. Example of poor storage of personal protective equipment on a shoe rack.

Figure 22. Lead aprons stored on a trolley and not laid flat—leading to creases and potential cracks.

Figure 23. Illustrates poor storage of a lead apron being used for mobile examinations.

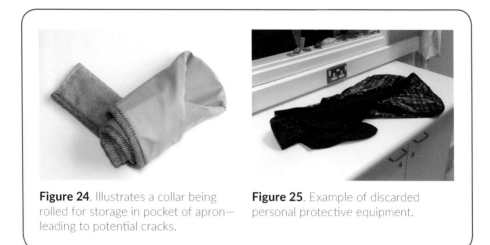

Figure 24. Illustrates a collar being rolled for storage in pocket of apron— leading to potential cracks.

Figure 25. Example of discarded personal protective equipment.

9.2 Cleaning and infection control

PPE should be cleaned according to the local infection control requirements. There should be an established program of regular cleaning.

In some clinical environments it is preferable to wear a plastic apron on top of the apron to make cleaning easier. To prevent damage to the coverings, only manufacturer-recommended cleaning agents and instructions should be used. It is not recommended to immerse the garments in cleaning agents. Sponging or gentle scrubbing should be adequate. Bleach may damage the coverings and reduce their life expectancy. Visible soiling should be cleaned immediately. Cleaning immediately after infective cases should be carried out as per the cleaning of all equipment with regard to local infection prevention and control policy. Some outer covers are more stain resistant and easier to clean than others and should be considered when purchasing.

Velcro fastenings often become "clogged" resulting in ineffective closure and should be "de-fluffed" regularly to maintain effectiveness.

Torn outer covers will present an infection control risk as they cannot be properly cleaned. If the cover cannot be repaired then the garment should be disposed of. Some suppliers will repair garments if they are not too old and this can be an economical alternative to replacement.

If possible keep a cleaning log and materials in, or close to the storage area.

9.3 Testing

It is important to perform specific quality control of protective garments.

Periodic testing of PPE integrity is an essential part of the quality control process since they are known to degrade over time, thereby compromising the level of protection afforded to the wearer. Degradation is strongly influenced by the frequency of use and the manner in which the PPE is stored between wear periods.

The Ionising Radiations Regulations 1999,[5] Regulation 10 states:

> "Every radiation employer shall ensure that all personal protective equipment provided pursuant to regulation 8 is, where appropriate, thoroughly examined at suitable intervals and is properly maintained".

All PPE should be checked to ensure there are no faults due to manufacture before it is accepted into service and then periodically re-inspected to ensure that no physical deterioration has occurred to compromise the effectiveness of the shielding. Since, anecdotally, it appears that the resilience of new "light lead" or lead-free materials may not be as good as traditional lead rubber, it is essential that all PPE is cared for correctly and regular monitoring of its condition is performed.

Records should be kept of the baseline and routine checks. All PPE should be given a unique identifier since it may be moved from one location to another. An inventory of PPE is a useful means of tracking, monitoring and identifying damaged PPE that needs repair or replacement and scheduling a replacement programme. If there are large numbers of PPE commercial software packages should be considered to assist in logging PPE.

A simple visual check for any signs of physical damage, particularly to fastenings, can be performed every time the PPE is worn. However, the damage is not always visible on the surface of the garment, as **Figure 26** illustrates.

A more thorough examination requires imaging the garment to detect holes, tears and variations in X-ray transmission. Reference to the examples of damage given below may help to prioritize areas to be tested. The damaged apron shown in **Figure 26** was detected during routine X-ray testing and taken out of use.

The testing should ideally be carried out using a fluoroscopy unit, where the operator can move the PPE and image as required, without manually repositioning the PPE. Where a department does not have access to this type of equip-

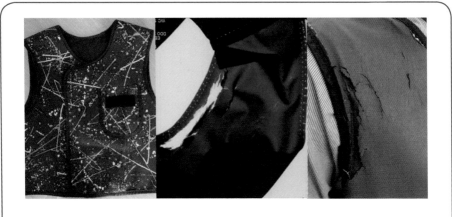

Figure 26. Vest shows no visible signs of deterioration (left image) but X-ray image (central image) reveals damage to protective material around right arm hole, which proved to be a 150 mm long tear in protective material and other damage, which is visible with outer cover removed (right image).

ment, assistance may be available from another facility. The use of mobile fluoroscopy is not recommended. In circumstances where fluoroscopy equipment is unavailable, radiographic checks can be made using conventional X-ray imaging, but care must be taken to ensure that the entire surface has been imaged and care also taken to minimize the manual handling.

The checks should be performed by two members of staff to reduce the manual handling risks from moving heavy PPE, especially if a number of aprons are to be tested in one session. The fluoroscopy equipment should be set on the lowest dose rate setting with the anti-scatter grid removed to keep the staff dose as low as possible. This is particularly important where remote fluoroscopy is not available. The PPE should be laid out flat and fully opened on the fluoroscopy table. The PPE should then be imaged over its entire surface in a systematic way. For wraparound aprons it may be necessary to adjust the position of the PPE to ensure it is completely screened. The staff performing the checks should have clear instructions on the rejection criteria in use in the department. An image should be stored of any damaged or suspect areas. These images can then be archived and reviewed by senior members of staff for a final decision on PPE that is borderline pass/fail. The stored image is also useful for ongoing monitoring of PPE that do not reach the rejection criteria but are showing signs of wear.

The interval required between more thorough examinations will depend on the type of PPE, the hazard against which it is required to protect, the conditions under which it is used, the likelihood of deterioration and the frequency of use.[6] The Guidance Notes[7] suggest that protective clothing should be thoroughly examined at least once a year to ensure that no cracks in the protective material have developed. The test period could be more frequent if there are any concerns about an apron that may have a small flaw that is acceptable but could deteriorate within the 12 month review period.

Thorough examination and testing will need to be carried out by people who are competent to do this work and in accordance with the manufacturer's instructions.

Example X-ray images of damage to PPE are given in **Figures 27–45**. It should be noted that it is normal to see stitching holes on X-ray images.

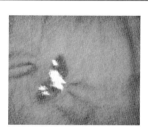

Figure 27. Damage assumed to be due to heat after leaving personal protective equipment kilt on a radiator.

Figure 28. Kilt damage probably due the garment being left folded or crumpled. This damage is slight, and depending on where it is this garment may still be usable.

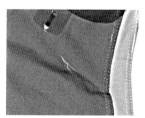

Figure 29. Small tear near shoulder.

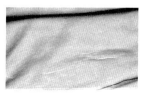

Figure 30. Fine cracks developed near edge of garment.

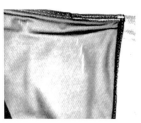

Figure 31. The cracks at the top of this kilt are probably due to the kilt being stretched at the waist fastener and/or the wearer being seated. Particular attention should be paid to this area on routine screening.

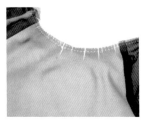

Figure 32. Small tears at neckline. These may make the garment very uncomfortable to wear and the tears may quickly become worse.

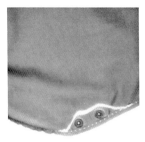

Figure 33. Damage around side clip fastening. This could be a result of the side clips being pulled too hard.

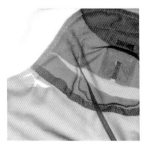

Figure 34. Large tear by apron shoulder fastener and small tear at neckline.

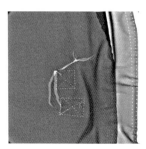

Figure 35. Tear around fastener.

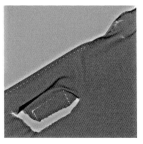

Figure 36. Tear at fastener.

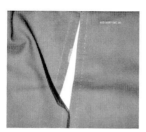

Figure 37. Kilt side seam has separated making it ineffective as a protective garment.

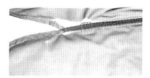

Figure 38. Apron material has separated from seam making it ineffective as a protective garment.

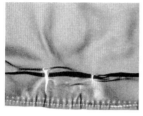

Figure 39. Damage to kilt at bottom back. The cracks have appeared where the protective layer has become creased. This may be due to heat or possibly just age.

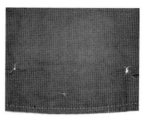

Figure 40. Damage to bottom of kilt.

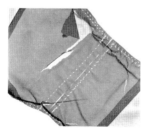

Figure 41. Apron shows significant deterioration, with separation of protective layers and a large tear at waist band and smaller tears elsewhere.

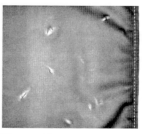

Figure 42. Small holes and other damage from scissors in back pocket of trousers.

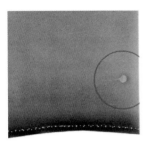

Figure 43. Coat hanger hole. Poor hanging meant hanger has gone through the apron.

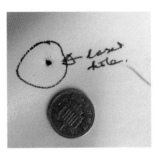

Figure 44. Photograph of laser entry burn damage to apron.

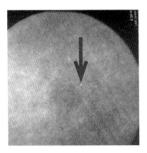

Figure 45. X-ray image of laser burn in **Figure 44**.

9.4 Rejection criteria

Any defects detected should be reported immediately and defective items should be taken out of use and replaced as soon as possible.

Decisions to reject PPE can be difficult. Some small cracks or holes may be acceptable especially if they are in areas of overlap *e.g.* where a top overlaps a kilt. In such circumstances it may be advisable to re-test more frequently to determine the stability of the damage. Record images if possible and mark the sights and extent of damage with a permanent marker.

In order to decide on actions to be taken, the important criteria are the size and location of any defects. Any holes or cracks in area of mid-line, breast, armholes, long bones and thyroid shields will probably mean rejection. As will torn covers that cannot be repaired.

The following criteria (**Table 2**) are intended only as a broad guide and specific advice should be sought from the Radiation Protection Supervisor and/or Radiation Protection Adviser. The criteria are based on the likely increase in effective dose to the wearer for varying levels and locations of damage.[49,50] It is recommended that PPE with defect sizes in excess of the rejection criteria should be removed from use immediately and replacement arranged if necessary. Any testing record should be updated to reflect the action taken.

Where "clearly not over a critical organ" means defects not in close proximity to radiosensitive organs,[15] or it is along the seam, or in overlapped areas, or on the back of the PPE. If the defect is clearly not over a critical organ and is <670 mm^2 then use of the lead apron may continue, provided the location of the defect is clearly marked on the lead apron and the size, location and date that the defect was identified logged in the apron quality assurance record.

Where multiple defects are observed in close proximity the overall total defect area should be estimated before applying the above criteria for rejection.

If the above table is used then it is suggested that local guidance also includes indications of the physical size of these areas *e.g.* discs of the appropriate size that can be laid alongside the defect for quick reference, taking into account any magnification factors in the image. For digital images it may be possible to use measuring devices on the imaging viewing system to determine the length/diameter of the damage.

Table 2. Outline rejection criteria for detected personal protective equipment damage

Location of defect		Maximum tolerable defect area	Maximum tolerable defect tear length
Lead apron	Over a critical organ	15 mm^2 (4.3 mm diameter circle)	20 mm
	Clearly not over a critical organ	670 mm^2 (29 mm diameter circle)	50 mm
Thyroid shield	Anywhere	11 mm^2 (3.8 mm diameter circle)	20 mm

9.5 Disposal

Where possible repair or redeploy garments if it is safe to do so.

The manufacturers of lead, light-lead and lead-free garments should state acceptable disposal routes. Most suggest that land-fill is acceptable for lead polymer and that incineration should not be considered as the fumes are toxic. Incineration or recycling is possible for some lead-free materials but the individual product information should be checked. Disposal options should be an additional consideration when purchasing PPE. The manufacturer's guidance and advice from the organizations waste management advisor should be followed.

Appendix 1. Quick reference table of SUGGESTED PPE requirements

The following table does not preclude the application of ALARP to an individual employee, but provides a suggested starting point for a risk assessment on PPE requirements.

Application	Annual whole body dose level (mSv)	Workload for individual employee (DAP)	Recommended apron (mm Pb eq)
General radiography	<2 (under PPE)	<1200 Gy cm²	0.25
General fluoroscopy	<2 (under PPE)	<1200 Gy cm²	0.25
Interventional radiology and cardiology	<2 (under PPE)	<50,000 Gy cm²	0.25
	<20 (outside PPE)		
CT interventional work			0.35
Operating theatre	<2 (under PPE)	<1200 Gy cm²	0.25
Dental radiography (operator)			None
Dental radiography (holding image plate or supporting patient)			0.25
Veterinary practice			0.25

DAP, dose area product; kV, kilovoltage; PPE, personal protective equipment.

Recommended thyroid collar (mm Pb eq)	Comments
None	Includes mobile radiography
None	If dose level or workload exceeded then thyroid collar recommended. If average kV exceeds 100, then 0.35 mm apron required
0.35	If dose level or workload exceeded then additional shielding or thicker apron recommended. If average kV exceeds 100, then 0.35 mm apron required
0.35/0.5	Assuming work is carried out at >100 kV
None	If dose level or workload exceeded then thyroid collar recommended
None	This assumes the operator can stand far enough away from the X-ray tube and patient during an exposure *i.e.* outside the controlled area. This should be defined in local rules. This does not apply to tomographic dental units
None	Applicable to staff keeping image receptor in place or supporting patient during X-ray
None	This assumes operator cannot stand far enough away from the X-ray tube and animal during an exposure *i.e.* outside the controlled area. This should be defined in local rules. If an animal is ever held then protective clothing may also be required for hand and forearm with lead equivalence of at least 0.5 mm

Appendix 2. Framework for PPE risk assessment

Department	
Area	
Type of work	
Work Load (potential staff dose per ???)	
How are employees monitored for dose	(under apron, outside apron, monthly, bi-monthly)
QA of PPE in place	Describe QA or reference procedure
Maximum KV for equipment covered by assessment	
Employees covered by assessment	Radiologist, Radiographer, Radiographic Assistant, Radiology Nurse, Other (list) [Delete any employees not covered by assessment]

Nature of hazard	Current actions	Current risk level[a]	Additional actions	Lead for implementation	Date completed	New risk level[a]
Incomplete protection due to poor fitting PPE	Variety of different aprons available to suit height and BMI range of staff		Purchase further styles/sizes of apron			
Incomplete protection due to incorrect wearing of PPE	Staff trained Posters on correct wearing in area Audit of employees wearing PPE					
Short operational life of apron due to incorrect care	Hangers available Employees trained on how to care for aprons Audit of care					
Injuries to back due to weight of apron and/or prolonged use	Ensure variety of aprons available Lumbar supports available Training of aprons Encourage staff to remove aprons between cases		Consider moving from 0.35 to 0.25 mm Pb apron provided thyroid collar worn, after discussion with RPA			

Date of Discussion with RPA	
Decision on what type of PPE to be worn	
Date communicated to employees	

References used to support decision on type of apron to be worn	
Name of assessor	
Grade of assessor	
Date of assessment	

Review date	Name of reviewer	Action required

BMI, body mass index; KV, kilovoltage; PPE, personal protective equipment; QA, quality assurance; RPA, Radiation Protection Adviser.
^aDetermine risk level using local risk management matrix.

References

1   The Personal Protective Equipment at Work Regulations 1992. Statutory Instrument 1992
     No 2966. London, UK: HMSO; 1992. Available from: http://www.legislation.gov.uk/
     uksi/1992/2966/contents/made

2   British Standard BS EN 61331-3 (2014). Protective devices against diagnostic medical X-radia-
     tion-Part 3: Protective clothing, eye wear and protective patient shields.

3   IAEA. Radiation protection and safety of radiation sources: International Basic Safety Standards.
     International Atomic Energy Agency, Safety Standards Series No. GSR Part 3. Vienna, Austria:
     IAEA; 2014. Available from: http://www-pub.iaea.org/books/IAEABooks/8930/Radiation-
     Protection-and-Safety-of-Radiation-Sources-International-Basic-Safety-Standards-General-
     Safety-Requirements

4   European Council Directive 2013/59/Euratom laying down basic safety standards for protection
     against the dangers arising from exposure to ionising radiation and repealing Directives 89/618/
     Euratom, 96/29/Euratom, 97/43/Euratom and 2003/122/Euratom. Official Journal of the Euro-
     pean Union 2014: 57. Available from: http://eur-lex.europa.eu/LexUriServ/LexUriServ.do?uri=O
     J:L:2014:013:0001:0073:EN:PDF

5   The Ionising Radiations Regulations 1999. Statutory Instrument 1999 No 3232. London, UK:
     HMSO; 1999. Available from: http://www.legislation.gov.uk/uksi/1999/3232/contents/made

6   HSE work with ionising radiation, Health & Safety Executive, Approved Code of Practice and
     Guidance L121. London, UK: HMSO; 2000. Available from: http://www.hse.gov.uk/pubns/
     books/l121.htm

7   IPEM Medical and Dental Guidance Notes. A good practice guide on all aspects of ionising
     radiation protection in the clinical environment. York, UK: Institute of Physics and Engineering in
     Medicine; 2002.

8   HSE personal protective equipment at work (second edition). Health & Safety Executive, Guid-
     ance on the Personal Protective Equipment at Work regulations 1992 L25. London, UK: HMSO;
     1992. Available from: http://www.hse.gov.uk/pubns/books/l25.htm

9   The Personal Protective Equipment Regulations 2002. Statutory Instrument 2002 No 1144.
     London, UK: HMSO; 2002. Available from: http://www.legislation.gov.uk/uksi/2002/1144/
     pdfs/uksi_20021144_en.pdf

10   Regulation (EU) 2016/425 of the European Parliament and the Council on personal pro-
     tective equipment and repealing Council Directive 89/686/EEC. Official Journal of the
     European Union 2016: L81. Available from: http://eur-lex.europa.eu/legal-content/EN/
     TXT/?uri=CELEX%3A32016R0425

11   The Manual Handling Operations Regulations 1992. Statutory Instrument 1992 No 2793.
     London, UK: HMSO; 1992. Available from: http://www.legislation.gov.uk/uksi/1992/2793/
     contents/made

12   The Management of Health and Safety at Work Regulations 1999. Statutory Instrument
     1999 No 3242. London, UK: HMSO; 1999. Available from: http://www.legislation.gov.uk/
     uksi/1999/3242/contents/made

13   British Standard BS EN 61331-1 (2014). Protective devices against diagnostic medical X-radia-
     tion. Part 1: Determination of attenuation properties of materials.

14   NCRP. Radiation dose management for fluoroscopically-guided interventional medical procedures. National Council on Radiation Protection and Measurements, Report No. 168. Bethesda, MD: NRCP; 2011.

15   ICRP. The 2007 recommendations of the International Commission on Radiological Protection. International Commission on Radiological Protection Publication 103. Ann ICRP 37(2-4).

16   Schlatti H, Zankl M, Eder H, Hoeschen C. Shielding properties of lead-free protective clothing and their impact on radiation doses. *Med Phys* 2007; **34:** 4270–80

17   Bateman L, Hiles PA, Parry AR. Comparison of lead and non-lead aprons. Proceedings of UK Radiological Congress 2006. Birmingham, UK. London, UK: British Institute of Radiology; 2006.

18   McCaffrey JP, Shen H, Downton B, Mainegra-Hing E. Radiation attenuation by lead and non-lead materials used in radiation shielding garments. *Med Phys* 2007; **34:** 530–7.

19   Jones AK, Wagner LK. On the (f)utility of measuring the lead equivalence of protective garments. *Med Phys* 2013; **40:** 063902.

20   Sutton DG, Martin CJ, Williams JR, eds. Radiation shielding for diagnostic radiology. Report of joint BIR/IPEM working party 2nd edition (2012). London, UK: British Institute of Radiology; 2012.

21   Marshall NW, Faulkner K, Clarke P. An investigation into the effect of protective devices on the dose to radiosensitive organs in the head and neck. *Br J Radiol* 1992; **65:** 799–802.

22   Martin CJ. A review of radiology staff doses and dose monitoring requirements. *Rad Prot Dos* 2009; **136:** 140–57.

23   Rawlings D, Faulkner K, Harrison RM. Broad-beam transmission data in lead for scattered radiation produced at diagnostic energies. *Br J Radiol* 1991; **64:** 69–71.

24   Tapiovaara M, Lakkisto M, Servomaa A. PCXMC: a PC-based Monte Carlo program for calculating patient doses in medical X-ray examinations. STUK-A139 (1997). Helsinki, Finland: Finnish Centre for Radiation and Nuclear Safety Authority; 1997.

25   Siiskonen T, Tapiovaara M, Kosunen A, Lehtinen M, Vartiainen E. Monte Carlo simulations of occupational radiation doses in interventional radiology. *Br J Radiol* 2007; **80:** 460–8.

26   HPA. Radiation risks from medical X-ray examinations as a function of age and sex of the patient. Health Protection Agency Report HPA-CRCE-028 (2011). Didcot, UK: HPA; 2011. Available from: **https://www.gov.uk/government/uploads/system/uploads/attachment_data/file/340147/HPA-CRCE-028_for_website.pdf**

27   Christodoulou EG, Goodsitt MM, Larson SC, Darner KL, Satti J, Chan H-P. Evaluation of the transmitted exposure through lead equivalent aprons used in a radiology department, including the contribution from backscatter. *Med Phys* 2003; **30:** 1033.

28   McCaffrey JP, Mainegra-Hing E, Shen H. Optimizing non-Pb radiation shielding materials using bilayers. *Med Phys* 2009; **36:** 5586–94.

29   Marshall NW, Faulkner K. Optimisation of personnel shielding in interventional radiology. In: Radiation Protection in Interventional Radiology. Proceedings of BIR–CEC meeting; 6 December 1993.

30 Rehani MM, Ciraj-Bjelac O, Vaño E, Miller DL, Walsh S, Giordano BD, et al. Radiological protection in fluoroscopically guided procedures performed outside the imaging department. International Commission on Radiological Protection Publication 117. Ann ICRP 2010; 40(6).

31 Pelz DM. Low back pain, lead aprons and the angiographer. *Am J Neuroradiol* 1999; **21:** 1364

32 Dragusin O, Weerasooriya R, Jaïs P, Hocini M, Ector J, Takahashi Y, et al. Evaluation of a radiation protection cabin for invasive electrophysiological procedures. *Eur Heart J* 2007; **28:** 183–9.

33 Maleux G, Bergans N, Bosmans H, Bogaerts R. Radiation protection cabin for catheter-directed liver interventions: operator dose assessment. *Radiat Prot Dosimetry* 2015. doi: http://dx.doi.org10.1093/rpd/ncv438

34 Cousins C, Miller DL, Bernardi G, Rehani MM, Schofield P, Vaño E, et al. Radiological protection in cardiology. ICRP Publication 120. Ann ICRP 2013; 42(1).

35 Stewart FA, Akleyev AV, Hauer-Jensen M, Hendry JH, Kleiman NJ, MacVittie TJ, et al. Statement on tissue reactions/early and late effects of radiation in normal tissues and organs – threshold doses for tissue reactions in a radiation protection context. ICRP Publication 118. Ann ICRP 2012; 41(1–2).

36 Barnard SGR, Ainsbury EA, Quilan RA, Bouffler SD. Radiation protection of the eye lens in medical workers – basis and impact of the ICRP recommendations. *Br J Radiol* 2016; **89:** 20151034.

37 Jacob S, Boveda S, Bar O, Brézin A, Maccia C, Laurier D, et al. Interventional cardiologists and risk of radiation-induced cataract: results of a French multicenter observational study. *Int J Cardiol* 2013; **167:** 1843–7.

38 Magee JS, Martin CJ, Sandblom V, Carter MJ, Almén A, Cederblad A, et al. Derivation and application of dose reduction factors for protective eyewear worn in interventional radiology and cardiology. *J Radiol Prot* 2014; **34:** 811–23.

39 Thornton R, Dauer LT, Altamirano JP, Alvarado KJ, St Germain J, Solomon SB. Comparing strategies for operator eye protection in the interventional suite. *J Vasc Interv Radiol* 2010; **21:** 1703–7.

40 McVey S, Sandison A, Sutton DG. An assessment of lead eyewear in interventional radiology. *J Radiol Prot* 2013; **33:** 647–59.

41 Van Rooijen BD, de Hann MW, Das M, Arnoldussen CWKP, de Graaf R, van Zwam W, et al. Efficacy of radiation safety glasses in interventional radiology. *Cardiovasc Intervent Radiol* 2014; **37:** 1149–55. doi: http://dx.doi.org/10.1007/s00270-013-0766-0

42 Martin CJ, Magee JS. Assessment of eye and body dose for interventional radiologists, cardiologists, and other interventional staff. *J Radiol Protect* 2013; **33:** 445–60.

43 Whitby M, Martin CJ. A study of the distribution of dose across the hands of interventional radiologists and cardiologists. *Br J Radiol* 2005; **78:** 219–29.

44 Whitby M, Martin CJ. Radiation doses to the legs of radiologists performing interventional procedures: are they a cause for concern? *Br J Radiol* 2003; **76:** 321–7.

45 Martin CJ, Whitby M. Application of ALARP to extremity doses for hospital workers. *J Radiol Prot* 2003; **23:** 405–21.

46 Reeves RR, Ang L, Bahadorani J, Naghi J, Dominguez A, Palakodeti V, et al. Invasive cardiologists are exposed to greater left sided cranial radiation. *JACC Cardiovasc Interv* 2015; **8:** 1197–206.

47 Uthoff H, Pena C, West J, Contrerasa F, Benenati JF, Katzen BT. Evaluation of novel disposable, light-weight radiation protection devices in an interventional radiology setting: a randomised controlled trial. *Am J Radiol* 2013; **200:** 915–20.

48 Martin CJ. Eye lens dosimetry for fluoroscopically guided clinical procedures: practical approaches to protection and dose monitoring. *Radiat Prot Dosimetry* 2016; **69:** 286–91. doi: http://dx.doi.org/10.1093/rpd/ncv431

49 Lambert K, McKeon T. Inspection of lead aprons: criteria for rejection. *Health Phys* 2001; **80**(Suppl. 2): S67–9.

50 Stam W, Pillay M. Inspection of lead aprons: a practical rejection model. *Health Phys* 2008; **95**(Suppl. 2): S133–6.

All website addresses are correct at the time of printing.

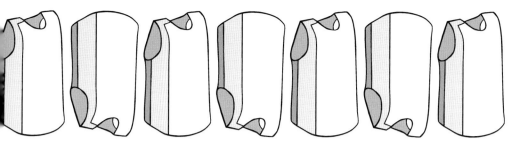

For more information and additional resources on

Personal Protective Equipment For Diagnostic X-ray Use

go to

www.birpublications.org/ppe

The British Institute of Radiology has produced a set of resources on PPE for staff working with radiation, to help develop radiation protection knowledge in and beyond the radiology department.

Book | Posters | Videos

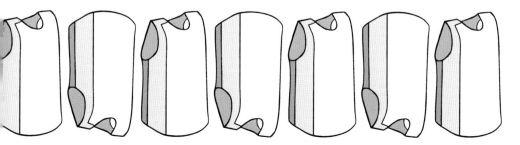